LOW HISTAMINE COOKBOOK FOR SENIORS

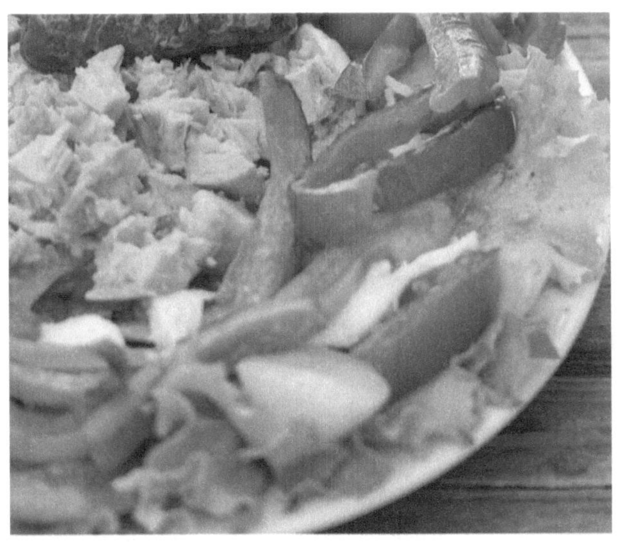

The Ultimate Guide to Prevent Histamine Intolerance With Tasty Gluten-Free Recipes For Older Adults

Lincoln Kimmons

Copyright © 2024 Lincoln Kimmons. All rights reserved.

How to Use This Cookbook

1. Start with Understanding: Become acquainted with the fundamentals of eating a low-histamine diet. Find out which foods to eat and avoid to properly control your histamine levels.

2. Plan Meals Mindfully: Make your weekly food plan based on the cookbook. Include a variety of recipes with an emphasis on fresh and minimally processed foods to guarantee a healthy and satisfying meal.

3. Shop Smart: Make a list of items to buy based on the recipes in the cookbook. When stocking your kitchen, go for items that are low in histamine, fresh veggies, and lean proteins.

4. Follow Recipes Carefully: Pay great attention to the cooking instructions in the cookbook. To stick to a low-histamine diet, follow suggested cooking times and ingredient substitutions.

5. Pay Attention to Your Body: Pay attention to how your body responds to various meals. Make changes to the recipes according to your tastes and any dietary restrictions. If necessary, seek medical advice to customize the diet to your particular health needs.

Remember that the secret is to enjoy the process of making the switch to healthier eating and not just follow the recipe exactly.

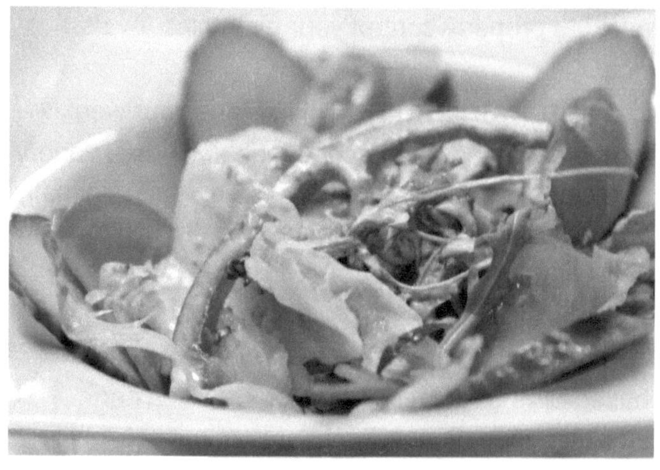

Table of Content

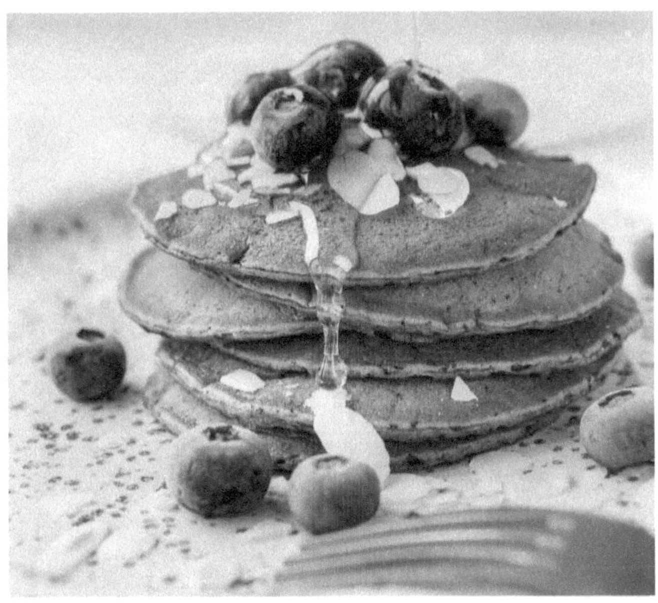

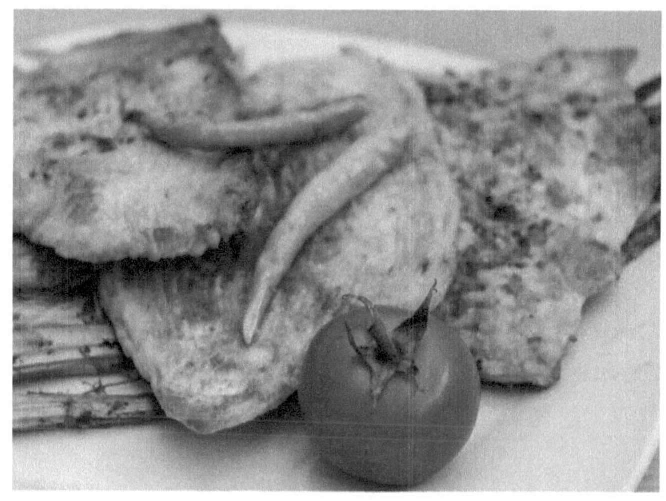

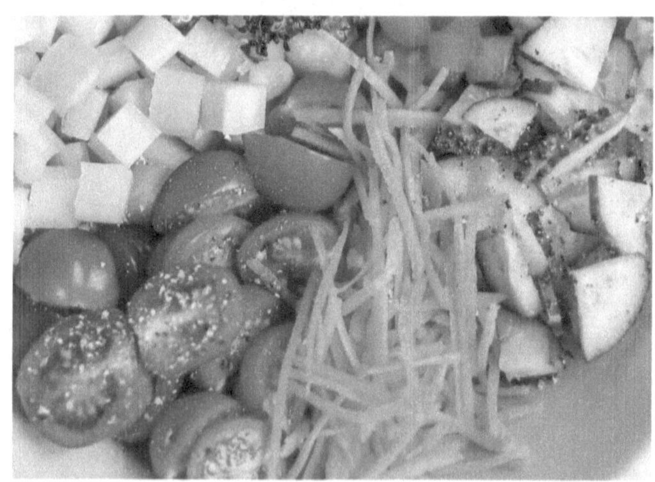

Introduction

Have you ever thought if a cookbook contains the key to regaining a tasty life? Imagine going on a journey where your kitchen becomes a happy place instead of a battlefield of food rules. This cookbook is more than simply a list of recipes; it's a roadmap to help you overcome histamine sensitivity.

A question lingers as you flip through its pages: does this cookbook hold the secret to opening doors to a world in which every meal is an occasion to celebrate health and well-being? The recipes are elegantly simple and incredibly delicious; they unfold like a culinary love letter, promising not just sustenance but also a symphony of flavors unhindered by histamine.

What if the solution to Emma's continuous health struggle lies in low histamine living? Exasperated by symptoms that failed to make sense, she set out to solve the riddles of histamine intolerance. Emma found a way to reduce her histamine levels and regain her newfound vibrancy and well-being when she adopted a diet and lifestyle.

The brilliance of this cookbook lies in its simplicity. As it avoids using unusual ingredients or intricate cooking methods. Simple components blend to create a happy, joyful space for cooking and culinary exploration in your kitchen.

With every meal comes a revelation: is it possible to transform meals into a celebration of health and happiness with a few well-chosen ingredients? The response comes back to you in the delicious results of your culinary endeavors, and it's a big "yes."

The cookbook serves as more than simply a reference; it becomes a traveling companion on your path to living a resilient life in which histamine intolerance is only one chapter. Another question comes up as you discuss your newly discovered gastronomic delights: Is eating a source of happiness and healing? The proof that it can happen is in the shared satisfaction after a wonderful meal and the laughter that occurs around the dinner table.

This cookbook is more than simply a guidebook; it's your reliable companion on your journey to a life in which each meal is a harmonious melody of well-being and joy.

Chapter 1

What is Low Histamine?

The body naturally contains histamine, which is used for several physiological processes. It serves as a neurotransmitter and is important for the immunological response.

When the body's histamine levels fall below the usual range, it is referred to as having low histamine.

Histamine is an essential substance that is involved in immunological responses as well as neurotransmission. People who have low histamine may encounter a variety of health problems since this imbalance might impair regular physiological processes. Dietary changes may be necessary to address low histamine levels because specific meals can affect the generation of histamine. Maintaining general health and well-being requires an understanding of and ability to manage low histamine circumstances.

Causes of Low Histamine

1. Diamine oxidase (DAO) deficiency:
DAO breaks down histamine. Histamine metabolism can be hampered by low DAO levels, which might result in symptoms similar to low histamine.

2. Certain Medications: Some treatments can lower the body's histamine levels and contribute to a low histamine state. Examples of these medications include antihistamines or drugs that inhibit histamine release.

3. Malnutrition: Low levels of histamine can result from inadequate consumption of nutrients such as vitamin B6, copper, and vitamin C, which are necessary for the synthesis of histamine.

4. Gastrointestinal issues: Disorders such as leaky gut syndrome or specific gastrointestinal conditions might impact the absorption of histamine and lead to reduced levels.

5. Genetic factors: Low histamine problems can result from rare genetic abnormalities that affect the body's capacity to manufacture or metabolize histamine.

Symptoms of Low Histamine

1. Digestion: Low histamine levels can result in gastrointestinal distress, including bloating, irregular bowel motions, and discomfort in the abdomen. These symptoms may be exacerbated by the lower histamine levels' effect on the control of stomach acid and digestive processes.

2. Skin issues: Inadequate histamine levels may have an impact on the condition of the skin, causing rashes, itching, or dryness. Histamine helps keep the skin intact, and a lack of it can make the skin less resilient to irritants, which may result in several dermatological problems.

3. Fatigue: Feelings of exhaustion and sluggishness may be caused by low histamine levels. Histamine regulates energy, and a lack of it might affect one's general vitality and attentiveness.

4. Headaches: Low histamine levels may be associated with ongoing or recurrent headaches. Headache symptoms may arise from disturbances in the blood vessel dilatation and neurotransmitter balancing processes, which are influenced by histamine.

5. Mood swings: Histamine interacts with neurotransmitters, and low amounts can aggravate depression or cause mood swings. Sustaining appropriate histamine levels is essential for the neurotransmitter activity balance in the brain, which impacts emotional health.

6. Allergies: Ironically, low histamine levels may increase an individual's sensitivity to allergens and thus their vulnerability to allergic reactions. The immune system depends on histamine, and a lack of it might affect the body's capacity to control and mitigate allergic reactions.

7. Joint pain: Some people with low histamine experience stiffness or pain in their joints. In cases of low histamine, these musculoskeletal symptoms may be influenced by histamine's role in immunological regulation and inflammation, albeit the precise processes underlying these effects are not entirely understood.

Preventive Measures of Low Histamine

1. Dietary Modifications: Include meals high in copper, vitamin C, and vitamin B6, among other nutrients that promote histamine synthesis. To control levels, also be aware of foods high in histamine and think about following a low-histamine diet.

2. Supplements: To assist histamine breakdown and metabolism, speak with a healthcare provider about suitable supplements, such as DAO enzyme supplements.

3. Hydration: Drink enough water to stay hydrated. Dehydration may exacerbate symptoms related to low histamine.

4. Gut Health: To improve nutrient absorption and maintain overall gut health, address gastrointestinal disorders with a balanced diet, probiotics, and lifestyle modifications.

5. Avoiding Triggers: Recognize and stay away from things like specific drugs and environmental triggers that can cause histamine to be depleted or make symptoms worse.

6. Handle your stress: Since stress raises histamine levels, learn stress-reduction strategies. Include routine-enhancing activities like deep breathing, meditation, or exercise.

6. Professional Advice: For individualized counsel, a diagnosis, and ongoing supervision for low histamine problems, consult a healthcare

provider. Collaboration with a healthcare professional and routine examinations are essential for properly managing and preventing symptoms.

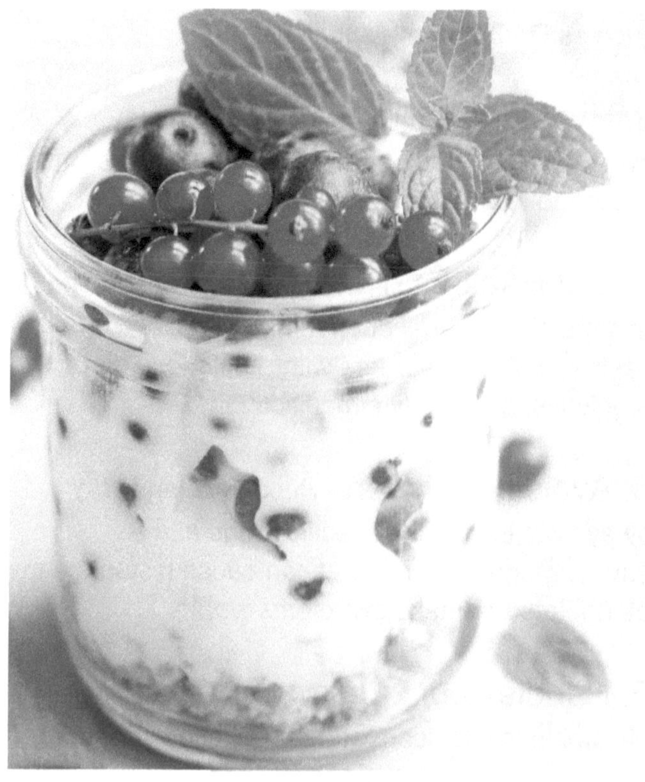

Chapter 2

Foods to Eat and Avoid

For those who are trying to control diseases linked to high histamine levels or who are suffering from histamine sensitivity, a reduced histamine diet is frequently advised.

Foods to Eat:

1. Fresh, Lean Meats: Choose lean meats that are freshly prepared, including fish, poultry, or turkey. In general, meat that has been freshly prepared has less histamine than meat that has been processed or cured.

2. Fresh Fruits: Histamine levels are often low in fresh fruits. Melons, pears, apples, and berries are all excellent options. Citrus fruits, however, should be used with caution as some people may have a histamine release.

3. Fresh Vegetables: You can add a range of fresh veggies, such as broccoli, zucchini, carrots, and leafy greens. It's imperative to choose fresh fruit and stay away from leftovers.

4. Pasta and white rice: It can be used as a base for meals and are generally well-tolerated. While some people may be able to manage whole grains like quinoa and oats, others may find that they induce histamine reactions.

5. Fresh Dairy Alternatives: Substitutes such as rice or almond milk are a good idea. It varies from person to person, although some people may be able to handle some cheeses.

6. Herbs and Spices: A lot of herbs and spices can enhance the flavor of food while being low in histamine. Turmeric, thyme, and oregano are a few examples.

7. Olive Oil: For dressings and cooking, use olive oil. When compared to certain other oils that can have higher histamine content, it is a healthier option.

8. Green Tea: Although both black and green tea have histamine liberators, people tend to handle green tea better. Individual reactions, however, could differ.

Foods to Avoid:

1. Fermented Foods: Foods that undergo fermentation may accumulate histamine. Limit or stay away from fermented foods such as pickles, sauerkraut, and soy sauce.

2. Aged Cheeses: Cheeses that have aged, like parmesan or cheddar, have increased histamine content. If you can tolerate cheese, go for fresher options.

3. Processed Meats: High histamine levels are seen in bacon, salami, and other processed meats. Select raw, fresh choices.

4. Some Fruits: While most fruits are safe to eat, some, including pineapples, strawberries, and bananas, might cause histamine release in people who are sensitive to them.

5. Vegetables High in Histamine: Some vegetables have greater levels of histamine, such as spinach, tomatoes, and eggplants. Exercise moderation may be required.

6. Canned or Foods Packaged: These frequently include chemicals and preservatives that raise histamine levels. Whenever feasible, choose to eat homemade, fresh food.

7. Alcohol: Wine and beer in particular can increase histamine levels. Compared to white wine, red wine often has greater levels.

8. Vinegar & Foods containing Vinegar: Although apple cider vinegar is frequently regarded as a good food, it has the potential to release histamine. Foods that have dressings or condiments made of vinegar have to be eaten with caution.

9. Chocolate and cocoa: Chocolate can react in sensitive people since it includes both histamine and histamine liberators.

10. Some Drinks: Some herbal teas, energy drinks, and carbonated drinks may include histamine or substances that release histamine.

Core Benefits of Following a Low Histamine Diet

1. Reduced Inflammation: As inflammation is a prevalent cause of age-related health disorders, seniors may find it easier to manage it with a low-histamine diet. Seniors who avoid meals high in histamine, which can exacerbate inflammation, may have less joint pain and feel better overall.

2. Digestive Comfort: Histamine intolerance can make gastrointestinal problems worse for seniors, who frequently struggle with digestion.

Eating a low-histamine diet can help with digestive comfort by reducing symptoms including bloating, abdominal pain, and irregular bowel movements.

3. Enhanced Energy Levels: Fatigue can be caused by imbalances in histamine, which is involved in energy regulation. Seniors following a low-histamine diet may feel more energized, which can facilitate an active and satisfying lifestyle.

4. Improved Skin Health: As people age, they frequently have skin-related issues. A low-histamine diet can help improve skin health by eliminating symptoms like dryness and itching by lowering potential triggers for skin concerns.

5. Improved Respiratory Health: Histamine affects respiratory function by playing a role in the body's reaction to allergens. A low-histamine diet may help seniors who have respiratory disorders since it may lessen symptoms associated with histamine and improve respiratory health.

6. Cognitive Well-Being: Disproportions in histamine can have an impact on cognitive function because of its interactions with neurotransmitters. A low-histamine diet may help seniors' cognitive health and may even lower their chance of cognitive decline.

7. Support for the Cardiovascular System: Unbalanced histamine levels and chronic inflammation can affect the cardiovascular system. By treating inflammation-related issues and encouraging a heart-healthy eating habit, a low-histamine diet may improve heart health.

8. Customized Nutritional Choices: As we age, our dietary requirements frequently change. Seniors can choose foods that are relevant to their health needs with a low histamine diet, which offers a personalized approach to nutrition.

9. Reduced Allergic Reactions: The sensitivity to allergens might be increased by histamine intolerance. Seniors may have fewer allergy reactions by eating a low-histamine diet, which improves their general comfort and well-being.

10. Joint and Muscle Comfort: A low-histamine diet may help seniors who suffer from arthritis or stiff muscles. By reducing histamine triggers, this dietary strategy may help relieve muscle and joint pain.

Chapter 3

How to Follow a Low Histamine Diet

1. Educate Yourself: It's important to know which foods are safe and which ones are rich in histamine before beginning a low-histamine diet. Typical foods high in histamine include aged cheeses, processed meats, fermented goods, and some vegetables. On the other hand, histamine levels are generally lower in fresh fruits, lean meats, and some cereals.

2. Create a Food Diary: Maintaining an extensive food journal facilitates tracking symptoms and identifying specific triggers. Keep track of everything you eat, and drink, and any symptoms you encounter. This can help you make necessary modifications to the low-histamine diet and offer insightful information on how your body reacts to certain meals.

3. Choose Fresh Over Processed: Whenever feasible, choose foods that are fresh and unprocessed. Histamine levels in fresh meats, fruits, and vegetables are often lower than in packaged or processed foods. Make cooking at home a priority so you can better manage the ingredients.

4. Pay Attention to Storing and Cooking:
Both of these processes might raise histamine levels in food. Meals that are made freshly are best, and leftovers should be quickly chilled. If you are preparing more food than you can eat in a short time, think about freezing portions.

5. Recognize and Avoid Trigger Foods:
Determine which specific foods can aggravate symptoms. Although broad guidelines exist, individual tolerance differs. If there are some meals that you find uncomfortable regularly, you might want to cut back on or avoid them.

6. Select Low-Histamine Proteins: Go for
fresh, lean meats like fish, poultry, and turkey. Histamine levels in these proteins are usually lower than in processed or cured meats. Steer clear of processed sausages, bacon, and other meat products rich in histamine.

7. Embrace Fresh Fruits and Veggies:
Make sure your diet consists of a range of fresh fruits and veggies. Leafy greens, zucchini, pears, apples, and berries are typically well-tolerated. But

exercise caution while handling spinach, tomatoes, and eggplants as they may contain greater levels of histamine.

8. Mindful Dairy Choices: Dairy substitutes such as rice or almond milk are better than conventional dairy. Since aged or fermented cheeses can contain more histamine, fresh cheeses can be a preferable choice.

9. Minimize Processed and Fermented Foods: Avoid pickles, soy sauce, and other fermented foods like sauerkraut. It is best to avoid eating processed and canned foods as they frequently contain preservatives and additives that raise histamine levels.

10. Track Symptoms and Make Adjustments: Continually evaluate your body's reaction to the low-histamine diet. If symptoms worsen or develop new ones, think about making more dietary changes or consulting a medical expert.

Healthy Shopping List

1. Fresh Meats: Select lean, fresh foods such as fish, poultry, and turkey since they often have

lower histamine levels than meats that have been processed or cured.

2. **Fresh Fruits:** Since they are often low in histamine, put berries, apples, pears, and melons on your shopping list.

3. **Fresh Vegetables:** Give leafy greens, carrots, broccoli, and zucchini priority. Vegetables high in histamine, such as tomatoes and eggplants, should be used with caution.

4. **White Rice:** White rice can be used as a foundation for dishes and is a well-tolerated grain. If you're following a low-histamine diet, think about adding it to your grocery list.

5. **Fresh Dairy Alternatives:** Consider using rice or almond milk as a fresh substitute. Fresh cheeses are preferably overaged or fermented if tolerated.

6. **Herbs and Spices:** A lot of herbs and spices can enhance the flavor of your food while being low in histamine. Add alternatives such as turmeric, thyme, and oregano.

7. **Olive Oil:** For dressings and cooking, use olive oil. When compared to certain other oils that

can have higher histamine content, it is a healthier option.

8. Green Tea: Although both black and green tea have histamine liberators, people tend to handle green tea better. If you're a tea lover, think about putting it on your buying list.

9. Fresh Eggs: Adding eggs to a low-histamine diet can be a flexible and nourishing option, as they are generally well-tolerated.

10. Nuts and Seeds: When making your grocery list, be sure to include fresh nuts and seeds such as chia seeds, sunflower seeds, and almonds. Individual tolerance, however, may differ.

11. Non-Citrus Fruits: Bananas and strawberries are examples of non-citrus fruits that are typically well-tolerated, although some citrus fruits have the potential to release histamine.

12. None- Histamine Fish: Opt for fish like haddock, salmon, or cod as they often have lower histamine levels than certain other seafood.

13. Fresh Herbs: You can add flavor to your food without overdoing the histamine content by using fresh herbs like basil, parsley, and cilantro.

14. Non-Histamine Grains: These include quinoa and oats, which have varying histamine contents but may be tolerated by some people.

15. Fresh Garlic and Ginger: In a low-histamine diet, both garlic and ginger are often well-tolerated and can give depth to your foods.

16. Homemade Broths: To reduce the amount of histamine in your broth, think about preparing your own at home with fresh ingredients.

17. Fresh Juices: Choose freshly squeezed fruit juices instead of concentrates or preservative-containing bottled juices.

18. Non-Histamine Sweeteners: Stevia and honey can be used as substitutes for processed sweeteners because they are often low in histamine.

19. Fresh Vegetables for Juicing: Use well-tolerated items such as kale, cucumber, and celery to make fresh vegetable juices.

20. Low-Histamine Snacks: For satiating and low-histamine snack options, try rice cakes, fresh fruit slices, and plain popcorn.

Complications of Low Histamine If The Right Diet Isn't Adopted.

1. Sleep Difficulties: It may be caused by decreased histamine levels, which are linked to the sleep-wake cycle. Those who don't make the right dietary changes may have trouble falling or staying asleep.

2. Impaired Wound Healing: Two critical elements of the wound healing process—inflammation and the immune system—are dependent on histamine. Low histamine levels can affect wound healing, which can cause injuries or surgical recovery to take longer to heal.

3. Hormonal Imbalances: The control of hormones can be impacted by histamine. If histamine levels are not controlled by food, people may suffer from imbalances in their hormones, which could affect other hormonal processes and reproductive health.

4. Increase Stress Response: Histamine interacts with the hormones that cause stress. People with low histamine may be more prone to an exaggerated stress reaction without following

the proper diet, which could result in elevated stress levels.

5. Respiratory Issues: Histamine plays a role in controlling respiratory issues. People may be more vulnerable to respiratory conditions like asthma or higher susceptibility to respiratory infections if their diet is not properly managed.

6. Nutrient Deficiencies: If the proper diet is not followed, certain nutrients, such as vitamin B6 and copper, which are involved in the metabolism of histamines, may become deficient. Widespread effects on general health and well-being may result from this.

7. Exacerbation of Pre-existing diseases: If histamine levels are not appropriately controlled by diet, people who already have pre-existing diseases, such as autoimmune disorders or chronic inflammatory problems, may notice an exacerbation of their symptoms.

8. Deficiency in Cardiovascular Health: Histamine plays a role in controlling blood vessels. People who don't eat a healthy diet run the danger of having their cardiovascular health impaired, which could result in problems like high blood pressure or circulatory disorders.

9. Enhanced Vulnerability to Infections:

Histamine plays a role in the body's defensive mechanism against infections. Without the right nutritional changes, people may experience a reduced immune system, which increases their susceptibility to infections.

10. Unbalanced Neurotransmitter:

Histamine interacts with many different neurotransmitters. Individuals who don't follow a healthy diet may have neurotransmitter imbalances, which could cause problems with mood, focus, and general cognitive function.

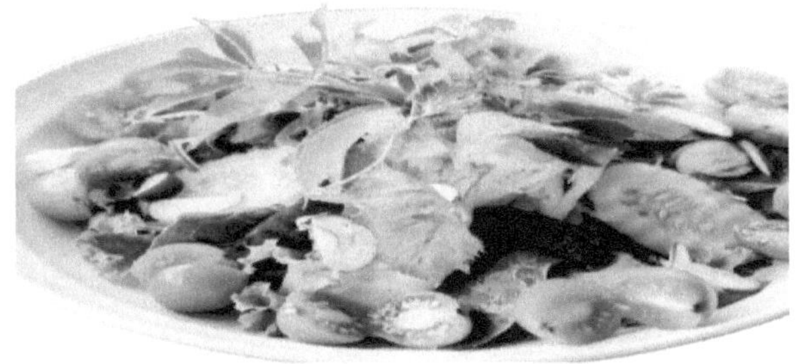

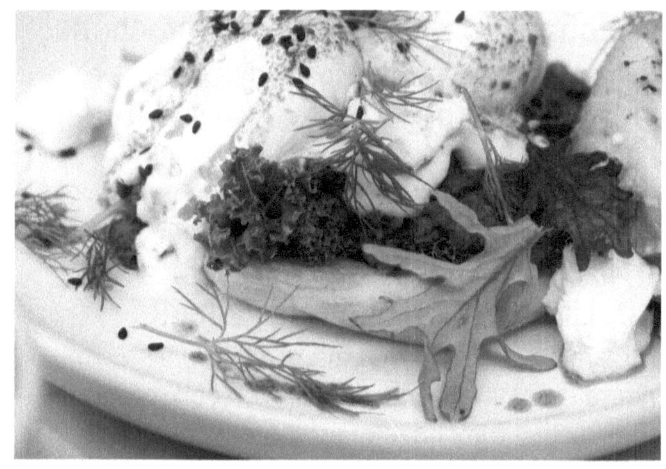

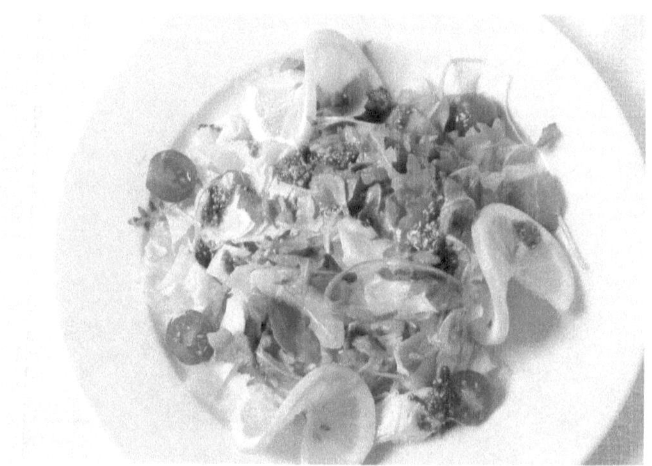

Chapter 4

Delicious Recipes

Breakfast

Quinoa Porridge

Ingredients:

- 1 cup quinoa (rinsed)
- 2 cups almond milk (or any milk of your choice)
- 1 tablespoon honey
- 1/2 teaspoon cinnamon
- 1/4 cup chopped nuts (e.g., almonds, walnuts)
- Fresh berries for topping

Preparation:

- Rinse the quinoa under cold water.
- In a saucepan, combine the quinoa and almond milk.
- After bringing to a boil, lower the heat to a simmer for fifteen minutes while covered.
- Stir in honey and cinnamon, then continue simmering for an additional 5 minutes or

until quinoa is cooked and the mixture thickens.

- Remove from heat and let it sit, covered, for 5 minutes.
- Fluff the quinoa with a fork and divide into serving bowls.
- Top with chopped nuts and fresh berries.

Nutritional Value (per serving):

- Calories: Approximately 350 kcal
- Potassium: 300 mg
- Sodium: 100 mg
- Protein: 10 g
- Phosphorus: 180 mg

Cooking Time: 20 minutes

Chia Seed Pudding

Ingredients:

- 1/4 cup chia seeds
- 1 cup of almond milk (or any preferred milk)
- 1 tablespoon maple syrup (adjust to taste)
- 1/2 teaspoon vanilla extract
- Fresh fruits (e.g., berries, banana slices) for topping

Preparation :

- Combine Chia seeds, almond milk, maple syrup, and vanilla extract in a bowl.
- To ensure that the chia seeds are evenly distributed, whisk the mixture thoroughly
- To avoid clumping, let the mixture remain for five minutes before whisking it again.
- Refrigerate the bowl for a minimum of two hours or overnight, covered.
- Before serving, stir the pudding to achieve a creamy consistency.
- Top with fresh fruits and serve chilled.

Nutritional Value (per serving):

- Calories: Approximately 180 kcal
- Potassium: 170 mg
- Sodium: 30 mg
- Protein: 5 g
- Phosphorus: 160 mg

Cooking Time: 2 hours (plus chilling time)

Spinach and Tomato Omelette

Ingredients:

- 2 large eggs
- 1/4 cup spinach, chopped
- 1/4 cup tomatoes, diced

- 1 tablespoon olive oil
- Salt and pepper to taste
- Optional: 2 tablespoons feta cheese (crumbled)

Preparation:

- Beat the eggs and season with salt and pepper in a bowl.
- Olive oil should be heated in a non-stick pan over medium heat.
- Add spinach and tomatoes to the pan, and sauté for 2-3 minutes until spinach wilts and tomatoes soften.
- Over the veggies in the pan, pour the beaten eggs.
- Allow the eggs to set around the edges, then gently lift the edges with a spatula, tilting the pan to let the uncooked egg flow underneath.
- Once the omelet is mostly set, sprinkle feta cheese (if using) over one-half.
- Fold the omelet in half with the spatula and cook for an additional minute until the cheese melts.
- Slide the omelet onto a plate and serve hot.

Cooking Time: 10 minutes

Buckwheat Pancakes

Ingredients:

- 1 cup buckwheat flour
- 1 tablespoon sugar
- 1 teaspoon baking powder
- 1/2 teaspoon baking soda
- 1/4 teaspoon salt
- 1 cup buttermilk
- 1 large egg
- 2 tablespoons melted butter
- Cooking oil for greasing the pan
- Maple syrup for serving

Preparation:

- In a large bowl, whisk together buckwheat flour, sugar, baking powder, baking soda, and salt.
- In a separate bowl, whisk together buttermilk, egg, and melted butter.
- Mixing until just mixed, pour the wet components into the dry ingredients. It's alright to have some lumps; don't overmix.
- Preheat a griddle or non-stick skillet over medium heat and lightly grease with cooking oil.
- For each pancake, pour 1/4 cup of batter onto the griddle.

- Cook until surface bubbles appear, then turn and continue cooking until golden brown on the other side.
- Take off of the griddle and continue with the rest of the batter.

Nutritional Value (per serving):

- Calories: Approximately 200 kcal
- Potassium: 180 mg
- Sodium: 300 mg
- Protein: 7 g
- Phosphorus: 120 mg

Cooking Time: 15 minutes

Greek Yogurt Parfait

Ingredients:

- 1 cup Greek yogurt
- 1 tablespoon honey
- 1/2 cup granola
- 1/2 cup mixed fresh berries (e.g., strawberries, blueberries, raspberries)
- 1 tablespoon chopped nuts (e.g., almonds, walnuts)

Preparation:

- Greek yogurt and honey should be thoroughly mixed in a bowl.
- In serving glasses or bowls, layer the Greek yogurt mixture, granola, fresh berries, and chopped nuts.
- Repeat the layers until the glass is filled, finishing with a layer of berries and nuts on top.
- Drizzle a little extra honey on the top if desired.

Nutritional Value (per serving):

- Calories: Approximately 300 kcal
- Potassium: 250 mg
- Sodium: 80 mg
- Protein: 15 g
- Phosphorus: 180 mg

No cooking required

Smoked Salmon Avocado Toast

Ingredients:

- 2 slices whole-grain bread
- 1 ripe avocado
- 4 oz smoked salmon
- 1 tablespoon cream cheese
- 1 tablespoon capers (optional)

- Fresh dill for garnish
- Lemon wedges for serving
- Salt and pepper to taste

Preparation:

- Toast the whole-grain bread slices to your preference.
- While the bread is toasting, mash the ripe avocado in a bowl and season with salt and pepper.
- Once the toast is ready, spread a generous layer of mashed avocado on each slice.
- Top the avocado with smoked salmon, ensuring an even distribution on both slices.
- Add a dollop of cream cheese on each toast and sprinkle capers (if using) over the salmon.
- Serve with lemon wedges on the side and garnish with fresh dill.

Nutritional Value (per serving):

- Calories: Approximately 400 kcal
- Potassium: 450 mg
- Sodium: 600 mg
- Protein: 20 g
- Phosphorus: 200 mg

Cooking Time: 10 minutes

Millet Breakfast Bowl

Ingredients:

- 1/2 cup millet
- 1 cup of almond milk (or any milk of your choice)
- 1 ripe banana, sliced
- 1 tablespoon chia seeds
- 1 tablespoon maple syrup
- 1/4 cup mixed nuts (e.g., almonds, walnuts), chopped
- Fresh berries for topping

Preparation:

- Rinse the millet under cold water.
- In a saucepan, combine millet and almond milk. Bring to a boil, then reduce heat to low, cover, and simmer for 15-20 minutes or until millet is tender and liquid is absorbed.
- Stir in sliced banana, chia seeds, and maple syrup. Cook for an additional 5 minutes.
- Remove from heat and let it sit, covered, for 5 minutes.
- Fluff the millet with a fork and divide it into serving bowls.
- Top with chopped nuts and fresh berries.

Nutritional Value (per serving):

- Calories: Approximately 350 kcal

- Potassium: 300 mg
- Sodium: 100 mg
- Protein: 8 g
- Phosphorus: 150 mg

Cooking Time: 25 minutes

Fruit Salad with Mint

Ingredients:

- 2 cups mixed fresh fruits (e.g., strawberries, pineapple, grapes, kiwi, mango), chopped
- 1 tablespoon fresh mint leaves, finely chopped
- 1 tablespoon honey
- 1 tablespoon lime juice
- 1/4 teaspoon vanilla extract
- A pinch of salt (optional)

Preparation:

- In a large bowl, combine the mixed fresh fruits.
- In a small bowl, whisk together chopped mint, honey, lime juice, vanilla extract, and a pinch of salt if desired.
- Pour the mint dressing over the mixed fruits and gently toss until well combined.
- Refrigerate the fruit salad for at least 30 minutes to allow flavors to meld.

Nutritional Value (per serving):

- Calories: Approximately 100 kcal
- Potassium: 200 mg
- Sodium: 10 mg
- Protein: 1 g
- Phosphorus: 20 mg

No cooking required

Vegetable Frittata

Ingredients:

- 6 large eggs
- 1/2 cup milk
- 1 cup mixed vegetables (e.g bell peppers, cherry tomatoes, spinach), chopped
- 1/2 cup shredded cheese (e.g cheddar, feta)
- 1/4 cup diced onion
- 1 clove garlic, minced
- 1 tablespoon olive oil
- Salt and pepper to taste
- Fresh herbs (e.g parsley, chives) for garnish

Preparation:

- Preheat your oven to 375°F (190°C).
- Heat olive oil over medium heat in a skillet. Add diced onion and cook until softened.

- Add mixed vegetables to the skillet and cook until they are slightly tender. Add minced garlic and cook for an additional minute.
- Mix the eggs, milk, pepper, and salt in a bowl.
- Over the veggies in the skillet, pour the egg mixture. On top, scatter the crumbled cheese.
- Cook for a few minutes on the stovetop, or until the edges begin to solidify.
- Transfer the skillet to the preheated oven and bake for 15-20 minutes or until the frittata is cooked through and golden brown on top.
- Garnish with fresh herbs before serving.

Nutritional Value (per serving):

- Calories: Approximately 200 kcal
- Potassium: 250 mg
- Sodium: 300 mg
- Protein: 15 g
- Phosphorus: 200 mg

Cooking Time: 25 minutes

Smoothie Bowl

Ingredients:

- 1 cup frozen mixed berries
- 1 ripe banana
- 1/2 cup Greek yogurt
- 1/4 cup almond milk (or any milk of your choice)
- 1 tablespoon honey
- Toppings: sliced fresh fruits, granola, chia seeds, nuts

Preparation:

- In a blender, combine frozen mixed berries, ripe bananas, Greek yogurt, almond milk, and honey.
- Blend until smooth and creamy. If necessary, add more milk to get the right consistency.
- Pour the smoothie into a bowl.
- Top the smoothie bowl with sliced fresh fruits, granola, chia seeds, and nuts.

Nutritional Value (per serving):

- Calories: Approximately 300 kcal
- Potassium: 400 mg
- Sodium: 80 mg
- Protein: 15 g
- Phosphorus: 180 mg

No cooking required

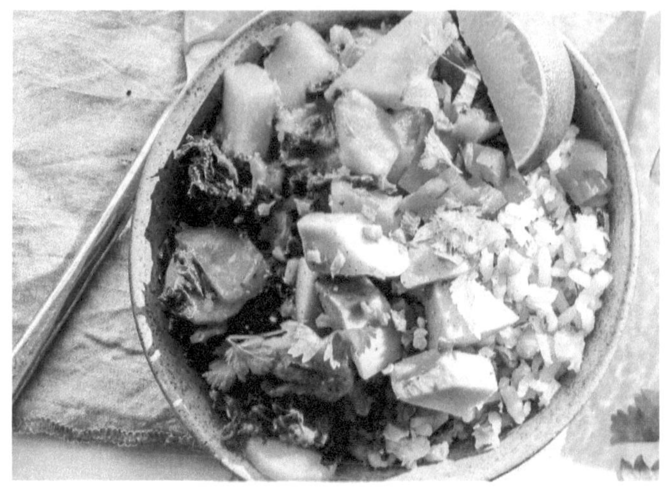

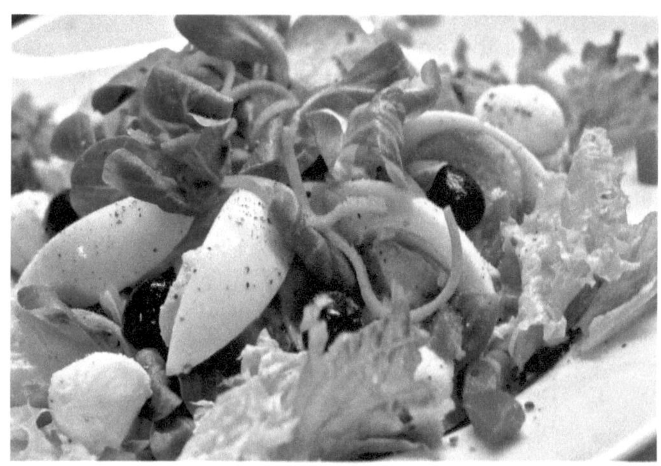

Chapter 5

Lunch

Grilled Salmon Salad

Ingredients:

- 1 lb (450g) salmon fillets
- 6 cups mixed salad greens
- 1 cup cherry tomatoes, halved
- 1 cucumber, sliced
- 1/2 red onion, thinly sliced
- 1/4 cup feta cheese, crumbled
- 1/4 cup Kalamata olives, pitted
- 2 tablespoons extra virgin olive oil
- 2 tablespoons balsamic vinegar
- Salt and pepper to taste
- Fresh lemon wedges for garnish

For the Marinade:

- 2 tablespoons olive oil
- 1 tablespoon lemon juice
- 2 cloves garlic, minced
- 1 teaspoon dried oregano

- Salt and pepper to taste

Instructions:

Marinate the Salmon:

- In a bowl, mix olive oil, lemon juice, minced garlic, dried oregano, salt, and pepper.
- Give the salmon fillets a coat of marinade and allow them to marinate for at least half an hour.

Grill the Salmon:

- Preheat the grill to medium-high heat.
- The salmon should be cooked through after grilling for 4–5 minutes on each side.
- Once done, let it rest for a few minutes, then flake it into bite-sized pieces.

Prepare the Salad:

- In a large bowl, combine mixed salad greens, cherry tomatoes, cucumber, red onion, feta cheese, and Kalamata olives.

Assemble the Salad:

- Top the salad with the cooked salmon.

Make the Dressing:

- Whisk together extra virgin olive oil, balsamic vinegar, salt, and pepper.
- Drizzle the dressing over the salad and toss gently to combine.
- Divide the salad onto plates.
- Garnish with fresh lemon wedges.

Nutritional Value (Per Serving):

- Calories: Approximately 400 calories
- Potassium: 700mg
- Sodium: 500mg
- Protein: 25g
- Phosphorus: 250mg

Cooking Time:

Marinating: 30 minutes

Grilling: 10 minutes

Assembling: 10 minutes

Quinoa and Vegetable Stir-Fry

Ingredients:

- 1 cup quinoa
- 2 cups water (for cooking quinoa)
- 2 tablespoons vegetable oil

- 1 onion, thinly sliced
- 2 bell peppers (any color), thinly sliced
- 1 zucchini, sliced
- 1 cup broccoli florets
- 2 carrots, julienned
- 3 cloves garlic, minced
- 1 tablespoon soy sauce
- 1 tablespoon sesame oil
- 1 teaspoon ginger, grated
- Salt and pepper to taste
- Sesame seeds for garnish
- Green onions, chopped, for garnish

Preparation:

- Rinse 1 cup of quinoa under cold water.
- In a saucepan, combine quinoa with 2 cups of water.
- Bring to a boil, then reduce heat, cover, and simmer for 15-20 minutes until quinoa is cooked and water is absorbed.
- Vegetable oil should be heated over medium-high heat in a large skillet or wok.
- Add sliced onion, bell peppers, zucchini, broccoli, and julienned carrots.
- Stir-fry the veggies for 5 to 7 minutes, or until they are crisp-tender.
- In a small bowl, mix soy sauce, sesame oil, grated ginger, minced garlic, salt, and pepper.
- Add cooked quinoa to the skillet with stir-fried vegetables.

- Pour the sauce over the quinoa and vegetables. Stir well to combine, ensuring the sauce coats the mixture evenly.
- Add chopped green onions and sesame seeds as garnish.

Nutritional Value (Per Serving):

- Calories: Approximately 350 calories
- Potassium: 450mg
- Sodium: 600mg
- Protein: 12g
- Phosphorus: 200mg

Cooking Time:

Cooking Quinoa: 20 minutes

Stir-Frying Vegetables: 7 minutes

Chicken and Vegetable Soup

Ingredients:

- 1 lb (450g) boneless, skinless chicken breasts, diced
- 1 tablespoon olive oil
- 1 onion, finely chopped
- 2 carrots, sliced
- 2 celery stalks, chopped
- 3 cloves garlic, minced

- 8 cups chicken broth (low-sodium)
- 1 cup green beans, chopped
- 1 cup corn kernels (fresh or frozen)
- 1 cup peas (fresh or frozen)
- 1 teaspoon dried thyme
- 1 teaspoon dried rosemary
- Salt and pepper to taste
- Fresh parsley for garnish

Preparation:

- Warm up the olive oil in a big pot over medium heat.
- Cook the diced chicken until It turns golden brown on all sides.
- To the pot, add the minced garlic, diced onion, sliced carrots, and chopped celery.
- The vegetables should soften after five minutes of sautéing.
- In a large pot, heat olive oil over medium heat.
- Add diced chicken and cook until browned on all sides.
- Pour in the chicken broth, dried thyme, dried rosemary, salt, and pepper.
- After bringing the soup to a simmer, cook it for 15 to 20 minutes.
- Add chopped green beans, corn kernels, and peas to the pot.
- Continue simmering for an additional 10-15 minutes until vegetables are tender.

- Adjust seasoning according to your preference.
- Spoon soup into bowls and garnish with fresh parsley.
- Taste the soup and adjust the salt and pepper according to your preference.

Nutritional Value (Per Serving):

- Calories: Approximately 250 calories
- Potassium: 600mg
- Sodium: 800mg
- Protein: 25g
- Phosphorus: 300mg

Preparing and Cooking Time: 40-45 minutes

Turkey Lettuce Wraps

Ingredients:

- 1 lb (450g) lean ground turkey
- 1 tablespoon olive oil
- 1 onion, finely diced
- 2 cloves garlic, minced
- 1 teaspoon ground ginger
- 1 red bell pepper, diced
- 1 cup water chestnuts, chopped
- 1/4 cup low-sodium soy sauce
- 2 tablespoons hoisin sauce
- 1 tablespoon rice vinegar

- 1 teaspoon sesame oil
- 1 head iceberg lettuce, leaves separated
- 2 green onions, sliced for garnish
- Sesame seeds for garnish

Preparation:

- Heat the olive oil in a big skillet over medium heat.
- Add ground turkey and cook until browned, breaking it apart with a spatula.
- Add diced onion, minced garlic, and ground ginger to the skillet.
- Sauté until the onions are translucent.
- Stir in diced red bell pepper and chopped water chestnuts.
- Cook for an additional 3-4 minutes until vegetables are tender.
- In a small bowl, mix low-sodium soy sauce, hoisin sauce, rice vinegar, and sesame oil.
- Pour the sauce over the turkey mixture in the skillet. Stir to combine and let it simmer for 2-3 minutes.
- Spoon the turkey mixture onto individual iceberg lettuce leaves.
- Add sesame seeds and sliced green onions as garnish.

Nutritional Value (Per Serving):

- Calories: Approximately 300 calories
- Potassium: 400mg

- Sodium: 600mg
- Protein: 25g
- Phosphorus: 250mg

Cooking Time: 15 minutes

Egg Salad with Avocado

Ingredients:

- 6 large eggs
- 1 ripe avocado, peeled and mashed
- 2 tablespoons mayonnaise
- 1 tablespoon Dijon mustard
- 1 tablespoon lemon juice
- 1/4 cup red onion, finely chopped
- 2 tablespoons fresh cilantro, chopped
- Salt and pepper to taste
- Bread or lettuce leaves for serving

Preparation:

- Put the eggs into a pot and pour water over them.
- After bringing to a boil, lower heat, and simmer for ten minutes.
- Transfer eggs to an ice water bath to cool. Peel and chop them.
- In a bowl, mash the ripe avocado.

- Add mayonnaise, Dijon mustard, lemon juice, chopped red onion, and chopped cilantro. Mix well.
- Gently fold the chopped hard-boiled eggs into the avocado mixture.
- Season with salt and pepper to taste.
- Spread the egg and avocado mixture on bread slices or lettuce leaves.

Nutritional Value (Per Serving):

- Calories: Approximately 250 calories
- Potassium: 500mg
- Sodium: 350mg
- Protein: 15g
- Phosphorus: 250mg

Cooking Time: 15 minutes

Baked Chicken with Herbs

Ingredients:

- 4 boneless, skinless chicken breasts (about 1.5 lbs or 680g)
- 2 tablespoons olive oil
- 2 cloves garlic, minced
- 1 teaspoon dried rosemary
- 1 teaspoon dried thyme
- 1 teaspoon dried oregano
- 1 teaspoon paprika

- Salt and pepper to taste
- Fresh parsley for garnish

Preparation:

- Preheat the oven to 400°F (200°C).
- Pat the chicken breasts dry with paper towels.
- Place them in a baking dish.
- In a small bowl, mix olive oil, minced garlic, dried rosemary, dried thyme, dried oregano, paprika, salt, and pepper.
- Apply an equal layer of the herb mixture to the chicken breasts.
- Bake in the preheated oven for 20-25 minutes or until the internal temperature reaches 165°F (74°C) and the chicken is golden brown.
- Before slicing, allow the chicken a few minutes to rest.
- Garnish with fresh parsley.

Nutritional Value (Per Serving):

- Calories: Approximately 250 calories
- Potassium: 350mg
- Sodium: 400mg
- Protein: 30g
- Phosphorus: 250mg

Cooking Time: Baking: 20-25 minutes

Mashed Sweet Potatoes with Green Beans

Ingredients:

- 4 medium-sized sweet potatoes, peeled and diced
- 1 pound (450g) fresh green beans, trimmed
- 2 tablespoons butter
- 1/4 cup milk (or non-dairy alternative)
- Salt and pepper to taste
- Fresh chives for garnish

Preparation:

- Place the diced sweet potatoes in a pot and cover with water.
- Bring to a boil, then simmer until sweet potatoes are fork-tender (about 15-20 minutes).
- Bring water to a boil In a separate pot
- Add green beans and cook for 4-5 minutes until they are crisp-tender.
- After cooking, drain and put the sweet potatoes back in the pot.
- Add butter, milk, salt, and pepper.
- Mash until smooth and creamy.
- Toss the cooked green beans with a little butter, salt, and pepper.
- Spoon the mashed sweet potatoes onto plates.

- Top with buttered green beans.
- Garnish with fresh chives.

Nutritional Value (Per Serving):

- Calories: Approximately 300 calories
- Potassium: 600mg
- Sodium: 150mg
- Protein: 4g
- Phosphorus: 100mg

Boiling Sweet Potatoes: 15-20 minutes
Cooking Green Beans: 4-5 minutes

Salmon and Cucumber Roll-ups

Ingredients:

- 4 oz (115g) smoked salmon slices
- 1 large cucumber
- 1/2 cup cream cheese, softened
- 2 tablespoons fresh dill, chopped
- 1 tablespoon capers, drained
- Zest of 1 lemon
- Salt and pepper to taste

Preparation:

- Wash the cucumber and cut it into thin strips using a vegetable peeler.

- In a bowl, combine softened cream cheese, chopped fresh dill, capers, lemon zest, salt, and pepper.
- Mix until well combined.
- Arrange slices of smoked salmon on a spotless surface.
- Over each piece of salmon, apply a thin layer of the cream cheese mixture.
- Place cucumber strips on top of the cream cheese.
- Carefully roll up each salmon slice with the cream cheese and cucumber inside.
- Place the roll-ups in the refrigerator for at least 30 minutes to firm up.
- Once chilled, slice the roll-ups into bite-sized pieces.

Nutritional Value (Per Serving):

- Calories: Approximately 180 calories
- Potassium: 300mg
- Sodium: 400mg
- Protein: 15g
- Phosphorus: 150mg

Assembling and Chilling: 30 minutes

Vegetarian Lentil Soup

Ingredients:

- 1 cup of dried green or brown lentils, rinsed and drained
- 1 large onion, diced
- 2 carrots, diced
- 2 celery stalks, diced
- 3 cloves garlic, minced
- 1 can (14 oz/400g) diced tomatoes
- 6 cups vegetable broth (low-sodium)
- 1 teaspoon ground cumin
- 1 teaspoon ground coriander
- 1 teaspoon smoked paprika
- 1/2 teaspoon turmeric
- Salt and pepper to taste
- 2 tablespoons olive oil
- Fresh parsley for garnish

Preparation:

- Rinse lentils under cold water and drain.
- Warm up the olive oil in a big pot over medium heat.
- In a large pot, heat olive oil over medium heat.
- Add diced onion, carrots, celery, and minced garlic.
- Sauté until vegetables are softened.
- Stir in rinsed lentils, diced tomatoes, ground cumin, ground coriander, smoked paprika, turmeric, salt, and pepper.
- Pour vegetable broth into the pot.

- Bring the soup to a boil, then reduce heat and simmer for about 25-30 minutes until the lentils are tender.
- Adjust seasoning according to your preference.
- Spoon soup into bowls and garnish with fresh parsley.

Nutritional Value (Per Serving):

- Calories: Approximately 250 calories
- Potassium: 700mg
- Sodium: 500mg
- Protein: 15g
- Phosphorus: 250mg

Cooking Time: 25-30 minutes

Tuna and Avocado Lettuce Wraps

Ingredients:

- 2 cans (5 oz/140g each) tuna, drained
- 2 avocados, diced
- 1/4 cup red onion, finely chopped
- 1/4 cup celery, finely chopped
- 2 tablespoons mayonnaise
- 1 tablespoon Dijon mustard
- 1 tablespoon lemon juice
- Salt and pepper to taste

- 1 head iceberg lettuce, leaves separated
- Cherry tomatoes for garnish (optional)

Preparation:

- In a bowl, combine drained tuna, diced avocados, finely chopped red onion, and celery.
- In a separate small bowl, whisk together mayonnaise, Dijon mustard, and lemon juice.
- Pour the tuna salad dressing over the tuna mixture.
- Toss all ingredients gently until they are well combined
- Season with salt and pepper to taste.
- Lay out iceberg lettuce leaves on a clean surface.
- Spoon the tuna and avocado mixture onto each lettuce leaf.
- Garnish with cherry tomatoes if desired.

Nutritional Value (Per Serving):

- Calories: Approximately 300 calories
- Potassium: 500mg
- Sodium: 400mg
- Protein: 20g
- Phosphorus: 200mg

Preparation Time: 10 minutes

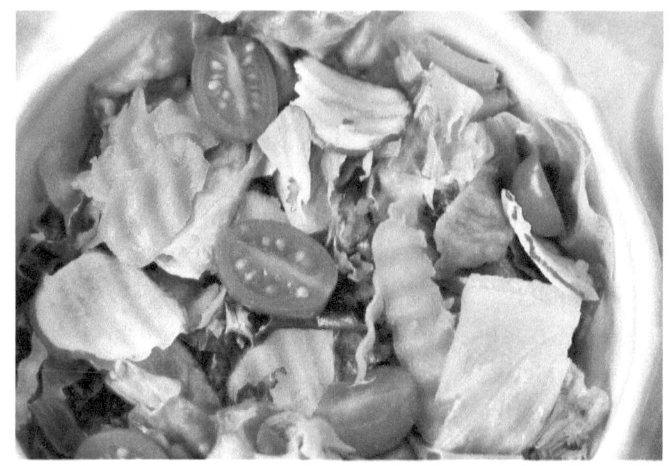

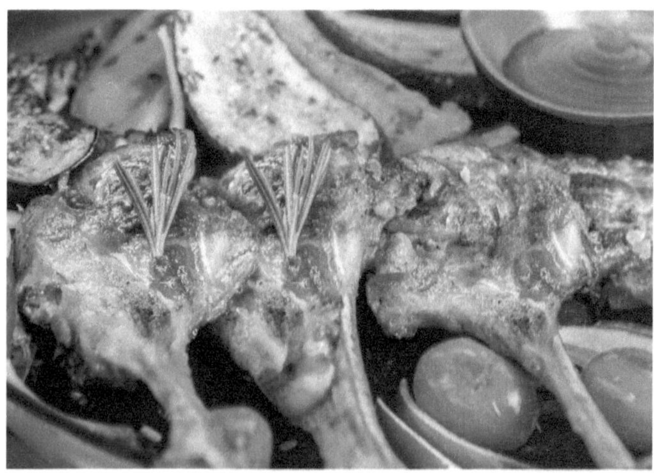

Chapter 6

Dinner

Lemon Herb Baked Chicken Thighs

Ingredients:

- 6 bone-in, skin-on chicken thighs
- 2 tablespoons olive oil
- Zest of 1 lemon
- Juice of 1 lemon
- 3 cloves garlic, minced
- 1 tablespoon fresh thyme, chopped
- 1 tablespoon fresh rosemary, chopped
- Salt and pepper to taste
- Lemon slices for garnish

Preparation:

- Preheat your oven to 400°F (200°C).
- Using paper towels, pat the chicken thighs dry.
- Place them in a baking dish.
- In a bowl, combine olive oil, lemon zest, lemon juice, minced garlic, chopped thyme, chopped rosemary, salt, and pepper.

- Make sure the chicken thighs are thoroughly coated by pouring the marinade over them.
- Let them marinate for at least 30 minutes.
- Place the baking dish in the preheated oven.
- Bake for 35-40 minutes or until the chicken thighs reach an internal temperature of 165°F (74°C) and the skin is crispy.
- Transfer the baked chicken thighs to a serving platter.
- Garnish with lemon slices.

Nutritional Value (Per Serving):

- Calories: Approximately 350 calories
- Potassium: 400mg
- Sodium: 300mg
- Protein: 25g
- Phosphorus: 250mg

Baking Time: 35-40 minutes

Salmon and Asparagus Foil Packets

Ingredients:

- 4 salmon fillets (6 oz/170g each)
- 1 bunch of asparagus, trimmed
- 2 tablespoons olive oil
- 2 tablespoons fresh lemon juice

- 2 cloves garlic, minced
- 1 teaspoon dried dill
- Salt and pepper to taste
- Lemon slices for garnish
- Fresh parsley for garnish

Preparation:

- Preheat your oven to 400°F (200°C).
- Cut four large pieces of aluminum foil.
- Place a portion of trimmed asparagus in the center of each foil piece.
- Each salmon fillet should be seasoned with salt and pepper.
- Place a seasoned salmon fillet on top of the asparagus in each foil packet.
- In a small bowl, mix olive oil, fresh lemon juice, minced garlic, and dried dill.
- Drizzle the lemon garlic marinade over each salmon fillet and asparagus portion.
- To create a sealed pouch, fold the foil over the salmon and asparagus.
- Ensure the packets are well-sealed to trap steam during cooking.
- Place the foil packets on a baking sheet and bake in the preheated oven for 15-20 minutes or until the salmon is cooked through.
- Carefully open the foil packets.
- Garnish with lemon slices and fresh parsley.

Nutritional Value (Per Serving):

- Calories: Approximately 350 calories
- Potassium: 700mg
- Sodium: 150mg
- Protein: 30g
- Phosphorus: 300mg

Baking Time: 15-20 minutes

Eggplant and Tomato Stew

Ingredients:

- 2 medium-sized eggplants, diced
- 1 onion, finely chopped
- 3 cloves garlic, minced
- 1 can (14 oz/400g) diced tomatoes
- 1 can (14 oz/400g) chickpeas, drained and rinsed
- 1 bell pepper, diced
- 2 tablespoons olive oil
- 1 teaspoon ground cumin
- 1 teaspoon paprika
- 1/2 teaspoon dried thyme
- Salt and pepper to taste
- 2 cups vegetable broth (low-sodium)
- Fresh parsley for garnish

Preparation:

- In a large pot, heat olive oil over medium heat.
- Add chopped onion and minced garlic, sauté until softened.
- Add diced eggplant to the pot and cook for 5-7 minutes until it starts to soften.
- Stir in ground cumin, paprika, dried thyme, salt, and pepper.
- To the pot, add the drained chickpeas and diced tomatoes.
- Mix well to combine with the eggplant and spices.
- Pour in vegetable broth, bring the stew to a simmer, then reduce heat and let it cook for 20-25 minutes.
- Taste the stew and adjust salt and pepper as needed.
- Ladle the eggplant and tomato stew into bowls.
- Garnish with fresh parsley.

Nutritional Value (Per Serving):

- Calories: Approximately 250 calories
- Potassium: 600mg
- Sodium: 300mg
- Protein: 8g
- Phosphorus: 150mg

Cooking Time: 20-25 minutes

Ground Turkey and Spinach Stuffed Bell Peppers

Ingredients:

- 4 big bell peppers, seeded and halved
- 1 lb (450g) ground turkey
- 1 onion, finely chopped
- 2 cloves garlic, minced
- 2 cups fresh spinach, chopped
- 1 can (14 oz/400g) diced tomatoes, drained
- 1 cup cooked quinoa
- 1 teaspoon dried oregano
- 1 teaspoon ground cumin
- Salt and pepper to taste
- 1 cup shredded mozzarella cheese
- 2 tablespoons olive oil
- Fresh parsley for garnish

Preparation:

- Preheat your oven to 375°F (190°C).
- After halves the bell peppers, remove the seeds and membranes.
- Place them in a baking dish.
- Heat the olive oil in a pan over medium heat.
- Add chopped onion and minced garlic, sauté until softened.
- Add ground turkey and cook until browned.
- Stir in chopped spinach and drained diced tomatoes.

- Cook until spinach wilts and excess moisture evaporates.
- Mix in cooked quinoa, dried oregano, ground cumin, salt, and pepper.
- Fill each bell pepper half with the ground turkey and spinach mixture.
- Top each with shredded mozzarella cheese.
- Cover the baking dish with foil and bake in the preheated oven for 25-30 minutes, then uncover and bake for an additional 10 minutes until cheese is melted and bubbly.
- Garnish with fresh parsley before serving.

Nutritional Value (Per Serving):

- Calories: Approximately 400 calories
- Potassium: 800mg
- Sodium: 400mg
- Protein: 30g
- Phosphorus: 300mg

Cooking Time: 35-40 minutes

Cauliflower Fried Rice with Shrimp

Ingredients:

- 1 head of cauliflower, grated or processed into a rice-like texture
- 1 lb (450g) shrimp, peeled and deveined

- 2 tablespoons sesame oil
- 1 onion, finely chopped
- 2 carrots, diced
- 1 cup frozen peas
- 3 cloves garlic, minced
- 2 eggs, beaten
- 3 tablespoons low-sodium soy sauce
- 1 teaspoon ginger, grated
- 2 green onions, sliced for garnish
- Sesame seeds for garnish
- Salt and pepper to taste

Preparation:

- Grate or process the cauliflower into rice-sized pieces using a food processor.
- 1 tablespoon of sesame oil should be heated over medium-high heat in a large skillet or wok.
- Add shrimp and cook until pink and opaque. Take out and place the shrimp aside from the pan.
- Add the last tablespoon of sesame oil to the same skillet.
- Sauté chopped onion and diced carrots until softened.
- Add minced garlic and cook for an additional minute.
- Stir in cauliflower rice and cook for 5-7 minutes until it begins to soften.
- Push the cauliflower rice mixture to one side of the pan.

- Pour beaten eggs into the empty side, scramble, and then mix with the cauliflower rice.
- Add the cooked shrimp and frozen peas to the pan.
- Stir everything together.
- Pour soy sauce over the cauliflower fried rice.
- Add grated ginger, salt, and pepper to taste.
- Garnish with sliced green onions and sesame seeds.

Nutritional Value (Per Serving):

- Calories: Approximately 350 calories
- Potassium: 600mg
- Sodium: 800mg
- Protein: 30g
- Phosphorus: 250mg

Cooking Time: 17 minutes

Baked Herb Chicken Drumsticks

Ingredients:

- 8 chicken drumsticks
- 2 tablespoons olive oil
- 1 teaspoon dried thyme
- 1 teaspoon dried rosemary

- 1 teaspoon dried oregano
- 1 teaspoon garlic powder
- 1 teaspoon onion powder
- Salt and pepper to taste

Preparation:

- Preheat the oven to 400°F (200°C).
- In a small bowl, mix olive oil, dried thyme, dried rosemary, dried oregano, garlic powder, onion powder, salt, and pepper.
- Pat the chicken drumsticks dry with paper towels.
- Brush the herb mixture evenly over each drumstick, ensuring they are well-coated.
- Arrange the drumsticks onto a parchment paper-lined baking sheet.
- Bake the chicken for 35 to 40 minutes, or until its internal temperature reaches 165°F (74°C), in the preheated oven.

Nutritional Value (per serving):

- Calories: Approximately 250
- Potassium: 300mg
- Sodium: 400mg
- Protein: 25g
- Phosphorus: 200mg

Cooking Time: 35-40 mins

Turkey and Vegetable Skewers

Ingredients:

- 1 pound (450g) turkey breast, cut into cubes
- 1 zucchini, sliced into rounds
- 1 red bell pepper, cut into chunks
- 1 yellow bell pepper, cut into chunks
- 1 red onion, cut into wedges
- 2 tablespoons olive oil
- 1 teaspoon dried thyme
- 1 teaspoon paprika
- 1 teaspoon garlic powder
- Salt and pepper to taste

Preparation:

- In a bowl, combine olive oil, dried thyme, paprika, garlic powder, salt, and pepper.
- Thread turkey cubes, zucchini rounds, red and yellow bell pepper chunks, and red onion wedges onto skewers.
- Brush the olive oil and spice mixture over the skewers, ensuring an even coating.
- Turn the heat up to medium-high on the grill or grill pan.
- After the turkey is well cooked and the veggies are soft, grill the skewers for 10 to 12 minutes, rotating them halfway through.

Nutritional Value (per serving):

- Calories: Approximately 300
- Potassium: 400mg
- Sodium: 350mg
- Protein: 30g
- Phosphorus: 250mg

Cooking Time: 10-12 minutes.

Mushroom and Spinach Quiche

Ingredients:

- 1 pre-made pie crust (9 inches)
- 1 cup (150g) mushrooms, sliced
- 2 cups (60g) fresh spinach, chopped
- 1 cup (100g) shredded Swiss cheese
- 4 large eggs
- 1 cup (240ml) milk
- 1/2 teaspoon salt
- 1/4 teaspoon black pepper
- 1/4 teaspoon nutmeg (optional)

Preparation:

- Preheat the oven to 375°F (190°C).
- Place the pre-made pie crust in a 9-inch pie dish.

- In a skillet, sauté the sliced mushrooms until they release their moisture and become golden brown.
- Cook the spinach in the skillet once it has been chopped until it wilts. Remove any extra liquid.
- Mix the eggs, milk, nutmeg (if using), salt, and pepper in a bowl.
- Spread the sautéed mushrooms and spinach evenly over the pie crust. Sprinkle shredded Swiss cheese on top.
- Pour the egg mixture over the vegetables and cheese.
- Bake in the preheated oven for 30-35 minutes or until the center is set and the top is golden brown.

Nutritional Value (per serving):

- Calories: Approximately 300
- Potassium: 350mg
- Sodium: 400mg
- Protein: 15g
- Phosphorus: 200mg

Cooking Time: 30-35 minutes

Baked Halibut with Tomato Salsa

Ingredients:

- 4 halibut fillets (about 6 ounces each)
- 2 tablespoons olive oil
- 1 teaspoon garlic powder
- 1 teaspoon dried oregano
- Salt and pepper to taste

Tomato Salsa:

- 2 cups (300g) tomatoes, diced
- 1/2 cup (75g) red onion, finely chopped
- 1/4 cup (15g) fresh cilantro, chopped
- 1 tablespoon olive oil
- 1 tablespoon lime juice
- Salt and pepper to taste

Preparation:

- Preheat the oven to 375°F (190°C).
- Place halibut fillets on a baking sheet lined with parchment paper.
- Drizzle olive oil over the halibut, then sprinkle with garlic powder, dried oregano, salt, and pepper.
- Bake in the preheated oven for 15-20 minutes or until the halibut flakes easily with a fork.

Tomato Salsa:

- In a bowl, combine diced tomatoes, chopped red onion, cilantro, olive oil, lime juice, salt, and pepper.
- Mix well and set aside.

Nutritional Value (per serving):

- Calories: Approximately 300
- Potassium: 450mg
- Sodium: 350mg
- Protein: 30g
- Phosphorus: 200mg

Cooking Time: 15-20 minutes

Shrimp and Zucchini Noodles

Ingredients:

- 1 pound (450g) shrimp, peeled and deveined
- 4 medium zucchinis, spiralized into noodles
- 2 tablespoons olive oil
- 3 cloves garlic, minced
- 1 teaspoon red pepper flakes (optional)
- Salt and black pepper to taste
- 1 tablespoon lemon juice
- Fresh parsley for garnish

Preparation:

- In a big skillet over medium heat, warm up the olive oil.
- When aromatic, add the minced garlic and red pepper flakes, if using.
- Season the shrimp with salt and black pepper and add them to the skillet.
- Cook until pink and opaque, 2 to 3 minutes on each side.
- Push the shrimp to one side of the skillet, and add zucchini noodles to the other side. Cook for 2-3 minutes, tossing occasionally until zucchini noodles are just tender.
- Combine shrimp and zucchini noodles in the skillet.
- Pour in some lemon juice, then toss to mix.

Nutritional Value (per serving):

- Calories: Approximately 250
- Potassium: 400mg
- Sodium: 350mg
- Protein: 25g
- Phosphorus: 200mg

Cooking Time: Approximately 10 minutes.

Chapter 7

Dessert

Blueberry Chia Pudding

Ingredients:

- 1/2 cup chia seeds
- 2 cups almond milk
- 1 teaspoon vanilla extract
- 1 tablespoon maple syrup
- 1 cup fresh blueberries
- 1/4 cup sliced almonds (optional for topping)

Preparation:

- In a mixing bowl, combine 1/2 cup chia seeds and 2 cups almond milk. Stir well to avoid clumps. Let it sit for 5 minutes, stirring occasionally.
- Add 1 teaspoon vanilla extract and 1 tablespoon maple syrup to the chia mixture. Thoroughly mix to distribute the flavors evenly

- Gently fold 1 cup of fresh blueberries into the chia mixture. Ensure the blueberries are evenly distributed throughout the mixture.
- Cover the bowl with plastic wrap or a lid and refrigerate the pudding for at least 4 hours, or preferably overnight.
- This enables the liquid to be absorbed by the chia seeds, giving the mixture a pudding-like consistency.
- To ensure a smooth texture and to break up any clumps, give the pudding a vigorous stir before serving.
- Optionally, top the Blueberry Chia Pudding with 1/4 cup sliced almonds for added crunch and texture.

Nutritional Information (per serving):

- Calories: Approximately 250 kcal
- Potassium: 200 mg
- Sodium: 50 mg
- Protein: 8 g
- Phosphorus: 180 mg

Preparation Time: 10 minutes

Chilling Time: 4 hours or overnight

Avocado Chocolate Mousse

Ingredients:

- 2 ripe avocados
- 1/2 cup unsweetened cocoa powder
- 1/2 cup maple syrup
- 1 teaspoon vanilla extract
- 1/4 teaspoon salt
- 1/2 cup almond milk
- Optional toppings: sliced strawberries, whipped cream

Preparation:

- In a blender or food processor, combine 2 ripe avocados, 1/2 cup unsweetened cocoa powder, 1/2 cup maple syrup, 1 teaspoon vanilla extract, and 1/4 teaspoon salt.
- Gradually add 1/2 cup almond milk while blending until the mixture reaches a smooth and creamy consistency.
- Taste the mousse and adjust sweetness or cocoa flavor if desired by adding more maple syrup or cocoa powder.
- Spoon the Avocado Chocolate Mousse into serving glasses or bowls.
- Refrigerate for at least 1-2 hours to allow the mousse to chill and set.
- Before serving, garnish with optional toppings such as sliced strawberries or whipped cream.

Nutritional Information (per serving):

- Calories: Approximately 200 kcal
- Potassium: 600 mg
- Sodium: 50 mg
- Protein: 3 g
- Phosphorus: 80 mg

Preparation Time: 10 minutes
Chilling Time: 1-2 hours

Baked Pears with Cinnamon

Ingredients:

- 4 ripe but firm pears
- 2 tablespoons honey
- 1 teaspoon ground cinnamon
- 1/4 teaspoon nutmeg
- 1 tablespoon of melted butter (or, for a dairy-free alternative, coconut oil)
- Greek yogurt or vanilla ice cream are optional for serving.

Preparation:

- Preheat the oven to 375°F (190°C).
- Wash and slice 4 ripe but firm pears in half. Remove the cores and seeds, creating a hollow space for the filling.
- In a small bowl, mix 2 tablespoons honey, 1 teaspoon ground cinnamon, 1/4 teaspoon nutmeg, and 1 tablespoon melted butter.

- Arrange the pear halves cut-side up in a baking dish.
- Spoon the honey-cinnamon mixture evenly over each pear half.
- Bake in the preheated oven for approximately 25-30 minutes or until the pears are tender and caramelized.
- Before serving, take them out of the oven and allow them to cool somewhat.
- Optionally, serve with a scoop of vanilla ice cream or a dollop of Greek yogurt for added richness.

Nutritional Information (per serving, without optional toppings):

- Calories: Approximately 120 kcal
- Potassium: 200 mg
- Sodium: 10 mg
- Protein: 1 g
- Phosphorus: 20 mg

Preparation Time: 10 minutes

Baking: 25-30 minutes

Coconut Yogurt Parfait

Ingredients:

- 2 cups coconut yogurt

- 1 cup granola
- 1 cup mixed berries (strawberries, blueberries, raspberries)
- 1/4 cup shredded coconut
- 2 tablespoons honey or maple syrup
- Mint leaves for garnish (optional)

Preparation:

- In serving glasses or bowls, layer 2 cups of coconut yogurt at the bottom.
- Add a layer of 1 cup granola over the coconut yogurt.
- Scatter a generous layer of mixed berries (strawberries, blueberries, raspberries) over the granola.
- Drizzle 2 tablespoons of honey or maple syrup over the berries for sweetness.
- Sprinkle 1/4 cup shredded coconut on top for added texture and flavor.
- Repeat the layering process until the glass or bowl is filled, ending with a layer of berries on top.
- Optionally, garnish with fresh mint leaves for a burst of freshness.

Nutritional Information (per serving):

- Calories: Approximately 350 kcal
- Potassium: 300 mg
- Sodium: 40 mg
- Protein: 8 g

- Phosphorus: 150 mg

Preparation Time: 10 minutes
Assembly Time: 5 minutes

Pumpkin Spice Rice Pudding

Ingredients:

- 1 cup arborio rice
- 4 cups whole milk
- 1 cup pumpkin puree
- 1/2 cup sugar
- 1 teaspoon vanilla extract
- 1 teaspoon pumpkin spice blend (cinnamon, nutmeg, cloves)
- 1/4 teaspoon salt
- Optional toppings: chopped nuts, whipped cream, extra cinnamon

Preparation:

- In a medium-sized saucepan, combine 1 cup arborio rice and 4 cups whole milk. Over medium heat, bring to a moderate boil, stirring occasionally.
- Reduce the heat to low, cover, and let the rice simmer for about 25-30 minutes, or until it absorbs most of the liquid, stirring occasionally.

- Stir in 1 cup pumpkin puree, 1/2 cup sugar, 1 teaspoon vanilla extract, 1 teaspoon pumpkin spice blend, and 1/4 teaspoon salt. Continue to simmer until the rice is tender and the pudding has a creamy consistency.
- Remove from heat and let the Pumpkin Spice Rice Pudding cool slightly before serving.
- Spoon into individual serving bowls.
- Optionally, top with chopped nuts, a dollop of whipped cream, and a sprinkle of extra cinnamon.

Nutritional Information (per serving):

- Calories: Approximately 300 kcal
- Potassium: 350 mg
- Sodium: 120 mg
- Protein: 8 g
- Phosphorus: 200 mg

Cooking Time: 35-40 minutes

Ginger Turmeric Smoothie Bowl

Ingredients:

- 1 frozen banana, sliced
- 1 cup frozen mango chunks
- 1/2 cup plain Greek yogurt

- 1 teaspoon grated fresh ginger
- 1/2 teaspoon ground turmeric
- 1 tablespoon chia seeds
- 1/2 cup almond milk (adjust for desired consistency)
- Toppings: sliced kiwi, pomegranate seeds, shredded coconut, granola

Preparation:

- In a blender, combine 1 frozen banana, 1 cup frozen mango chunks, 1/2 cup plain Greek yogurt, 1 teaspoon grated fresh ginger, 1/2 teaspoon ground turmeric, 1 tablespoon chia seeds, and 1/2 cup almond milk.
- To get the right consistency, add extra almond milk if necessary and blend until smooth and creamy.
- Pour the ginger turmeric smoothie into a bowl.
- Top with sliced kiwi, pomegranate seeds, shredded coconut, and granola for added texture and flavor.
- For added sweetness, feel free to sprinkle with honey or maple syrup.

Nutritional Information (per serving):

- Calories: Approximately 350 kcal
- Potassium: 800 mg
- Sodium: 70 mg

- Protein: 15 g
- Phosphorus: 250 mg

Preparation Time: 7 minutes

Almond Butter Banana Bites

Ingredients:

- 2 large bananas, peeled and sliced into 1-inch rounds
- 1/4 cup almond butter
- 1/4 cup granola
- 2 tablespoons honey
- 2 tablespoons chopped almonds

Preparation:

- Arrange the slices of banana on a tray or dish.
- Spread a small amount of almond butter on top of each banana slice.
- Sprinkle granola evenly over the almond butter-covered banana slices.
- Drizzle each banana bite with a touch of honey for sweetness.
- Top each bite with chopped almonds for added crunch.
- Serve immediately or refrigerate for a refreshing and satisfying snack.

Nutritional value (per serving, based on 4 servings):

- Calories: Approximately 150 kcal
- Potassium: 300 mg
- Sodium: 10 mg
- Protein: 3 g
- Phosphorus: 80 mg

Preparation Time: 10 minutes

Vanilla Berry Sorbet

Ingredients:

- 3 cups mixed berries (strawberries, blueberries, raspberries)
- 1/2 cup granulated sugar
- 1 tablespoon lemon juice
- 1 teaspoon vanilla extract
- 1 cup water

Preparation:

- In a saucepan, combine 3 cups mixed berries, 1/2 cup granulated sugar, 1 tablespoon lemon juice, and 1 cup water.
- Over medium heat, bring the mixture to a moderate boil.

- Stir occasionally and let it simmer for about 5-7 minutes until the berries are soft and the sugar is dissolved.
- After taking the mixture off the heat, let it cool to room temperature.
- After the berry mixture has cooled, move it to a food processor or blender.
- Add 1 teaspoon vanilla extract to the blender and blend until smooth.
- Pour the mixture into a shallow dish and freeze for 4-6 hours, or until it reaches a sorbet consistency.
- Every hour, stir the sorbet with a fork to break up ice crystals and ensure a smooth texture.
- Once fully frozen and firm, scoop the Vanilla Berry Sorbet into serving bowls.

Nutritional Information (per serving, based on 4 servings):

- Calories: Approximately 120 kcal
- Potassium: 150 mg
- Sodium: 5 mg
- Protein: 1 g
- Phosphorus: 30 mg

Preparation Time: 10 minutes

Freezing Time: 4-6 hours

Quinoa Apple Crisp

Ingredients:

For the Filling:

- 4 large apples, peeled and thinly sliced
- 2 tablespoons maple syrup
- 1 teaspoon ground cinnamon
- 1 tablespoon lemon juice
- 1 tablespoon all-purpose flour

For the Crisp Topping:

- 1 cup cooked quinoa
- 1/2 cup old-fashioned rolled oats
- 1/4 cup almond flour
- 1/4 cup chopped walnuts or pecans
- 1/4 cup melted coconut oil
- 2 tablespoons maple syrup
- 1 teaspoon vanilla extract
- 1/2 teaspoon ground cinnamon
- 1/4 teaspoon salt

Preparation:

- Preheat the oven to 350°F (175°C).
- In a large bowl, combine the sliced apples with 2 tablespoons of maple syrup, 1 teaspoon ground cinnamon, 1 tablespoon lemon juice, and 1 tablespoon all-purpose

flour. Toss the apples until they are coated all over.

- In a separate bowl, mix the cooked quinoa, rolled oats, almond flour, chopped nuts, melted coconut oil, maple syrup, vanilla extract, cinnamon, and salt. This creates a crisp topping.
- Grease a baking dish and spread the apple mixture evenly at the bottom.
- Sprinkle the quinoa-oat topping over the apples, covering them completely.
- Bake in the preheated oven for 35-40 minutes or until the top is golden brown and the apples are tender.
- Allow the Quinoa Apple Crisp to cool for a few minutes before serving.

Nutritional Information (per serving, based on 6 servings):

- Calories: Approximately 300 kcal
- Potassium: 250 mg
- Sodium: 50 mg
- Protein: 5 g
- Phosphorus: 100 mg

Preparation Time: 20 minutes

Baking Time: 35-40 minutes

Mango Mint Sorbet

Ingredients:

- 1 cup ripe mango, diced
- 2 tablespoons fresh mint leaves
- 2 tablespoons granulated sugar
- 1/2 tablespoon lime juice
- 2 tablespoons water

Preparation:

- In a blender, combine 1 cup diced ripe mango, 2 tablespoons fresh mint leaves, 2 tablespoons granulated sugar, 1/2 tablespoon lime juice, and 2 tablespoons water.
- Blend until smooth and well combined.
- Taste the mixture and adjust sweetness or mint flavor if necessary.
- Pour the sorbet mixture into a shallow dish and freeze for 4-6 hours or until it reaches a sorbet consistency.
- Every hour, stir the sorbet with a fork to break up ice crystals and maintain a smooth texture.
- Once the Mango Mint Sorbet is fully frozen, scoop it into serving bowls.

Nutritional Information (per serving):

- Calories: Approximately 60 kcal

- Potassium: 75 mg
- Sodium: 3 mg
- Protein: 0.5 g
- Phosphorus: 10 mg

Preparation Time: 10 minutes

Freezing Time: 4-6 hours

Conclusion

In conclusion, this cookbook is akin to a recipe book for delicious, healthful meals that are appropriate for senior citizens who are low in histamine. It's all about avoiding meals high in histamine, which can be problematic for the body systems as you age and utilizing fresh, minimally processed items.

Not only are the meals healthy, but they taste amazing. Additionally, they include anti-inflammatory ingredients to further improve your overall health.

So what use is all of this? Trying these dishes is like taking control of your health, aside from the fact that they will make you feel better physically. It's about feeling strong and well into old age, not just about what you consume.

Consider this to be more than just cooking as you work through these dishes. Saying "Hey, I care about myself, and I'm going to enjoy every bite of it!" is what it means. It's like giving yourself the gift of feeling amazing when you incorporate this low-histamine diet into your daily routine. Together, let's liven it up with delicious cuisine that loves your body back!

Bonus

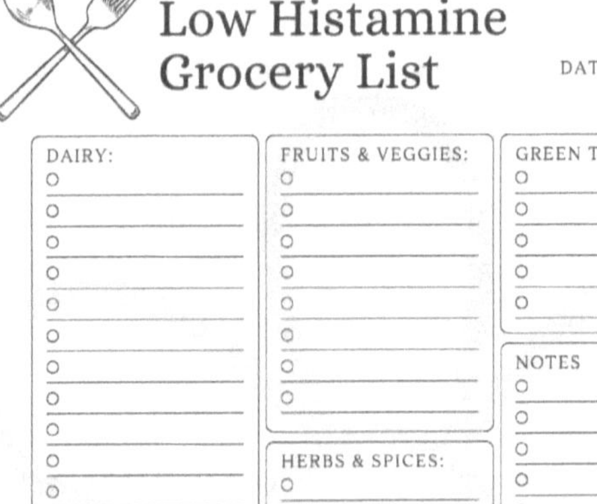

DAIRY:

FRUITS & VEGGIES:

GREEN TEA

NOTES

HERBS & SPICES:

MEAT & SEAFOOD:

OTHERS:

WHAT'S FOR TODAY

S
M
T
W
T
F
S

Low Histamine
Grocery List

DATE:

DAIRY:
-
-
-
-
-
-
-
-
-
-
-
-

MEAT & SEAFOOD:
-
-
-
-
-
-
-
-
-
-
-
-

FRUITS & VEGGIES:
-
-
-
-
-
-
-
-

HERBS & SPICES:
-
-
-
-
-

OTHERS:
-
-
-
-
-
-
-
-

GREEN TEA
-
-
-
-
-

NOTES
-
-
-
-
-

WHAT'S FOR TODAY
- S
- M
- T
- W
- T
- F
- S

Low Histamine Grocery List

DATE:

DAIRY:

FRUITS & VEGGIES:

GREEN TEA

NOTES

HERBS & SPICES:

MEAT & SEAFOOD:

OTHERS:

WHAT'S FOR TODAY

S
M
T
W
T
F
S

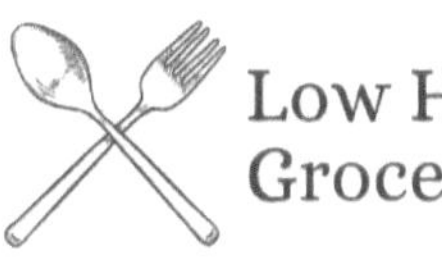

Low Histamine
Grocery List

DATE:

DAIRY:

FRUITS & VEGGIES:

GREEN TEA

NOTES

HERBS & SPICES:

MEAT & SEAFOOD:

OTHERS:

WHAT'S FOR TODAY

S

M

T

W

T

F

S

Low Histamine Grocery List

DATE:

DAIRY:
- ○ _______________
- ○ _______________
- ○ _______________
- ○ _______________
- ○ _______________
- ○ _______________
- ○ _______________
- ○ _______________
- ○ _______________
- ○ _______________
- ○ _______________
- ○ _______________

MEAT & SEAFOOD:
- ○ _______________
- ○ _______________
- ○ _______________
- ○ _______________
- ○ _______________
- ○ _______________
- ○ _______________
- ○ _______________
- ○ _______________
- ○ _______________
- ○ _______________
- ○ _______________
- ○ _______________

FRUITS & VEGGIES:
- ○ _______________
- ○ _______________
- ○ _______________
- ○ _______________
- ○ _______________
- ○ _______________
- ○ _______________
- ○ _______________

HERBS & SPICES:
- ○ _______________
- ○ _______________
- ○ _______________
- ○ _______________
- ○ _______________

OTHERS:
- ○ _______________
- ○ _______________
- ○ _______________
- ○ _______________
- ○ _______________
- ○ _______________
- ○ _______________
- ○ _______________

GREEN TEA
- ○ _______________
- ○ _______________
- ○ _______________
- ○ _______________
- ○ _______________

NOTES
- ○ _______________
- ○ _______________
- ○ _______________
- ○ _______________
- ○ _______________

WHAT'S FOR TODAY
- S
- M
- T
- W
- T
- F
- S

Low Histamine Grocery List

DATE:

DAIRY:
- ○
- ○
- ○
- ○
- ○
- ○
- ○
- ○
- ○
- ○
- ○
- ○

MEAT & SEAFOOD:
- ○
- ○
- ○
- ○
- ○
- ○
- ○
- ○
- ○
- ○
- ○
- ○

FRUITS & VEGGIES:
- ○
- ○
- ○
- ○
- ○
- ○
- ○
- ○

HERBS & SPICES:
- ○
- ○
- ○
- ○
- ○

OTHERS:
- ○
- ○
- ○
- ○
- ○
- ○
- ○
- ○

GREEN TEA
- ○
- ○
- ○
- ○
- ○

NOTES
- ○
- ○
- ○
- ○
- ○

WHAT'S FOR TODAY
- S
- M
- T
- W
- T
- F
- S

Low Histamine Grocery List

DATE:

DAIRY:
-
-
-
-
-
-
-
-
-
-
-
-

MEAT & SEAFOOD:
-
-
-
-
-
-
-
-
-
-
-
-

FRUITS & VEGGIES:
-
-
-
-
-
-
-
-

HERBS & SPICES:
-
-
-
-
-

OTHERS:
-
-
-
-
-
-
-
-

GREEN TEA
-
-
-
-
-

NOTES
-
-
-
-
-

WHAT'S FOR TODAY

- S
- M
- T
- W
- T
- F
- S

Low Histamine
Grocery List

DATE:

DAIRY:
- ○
- ○
- ○
- ○
- ○
- ○
- ○
- ○
- ○
- ○
- ○
- ○

MEAT & SEAFOOD:
- ○
- ○
- ○
- ○
- ○
- ○
- ○
- ○
- ○
- ○
- ○
- ○

FRUITS & VEGGIES:
- ○
- ○
- ○
- ○
- ○
- ○
- ○

HERBS & SPICES:
- ○
- ○
- ○
- ○
- ○

OTHERS:
- ○
- ○
- ○
- ○
- ○
- ○
- ○
- ○

GREEN TEA
- ○
- ○
- ○
- ○
- ○

NOTES
- ○
- ○
- ○
- ○
- ○

WHAT'S FOR TODAY

S

M

T

W

T

F

S

Low Histamine Grocery List

DATE:

DAIRY:

FRUITS & VEGGIES:

GREEN TEA

NOTES

HERBS & SPICES:

MEAT & SEAFOOD:

OTHERS:

WHAT'S FOR TODAY

S

M

T

W

T

F

S

Low Histamine Grocery List

DATE:

DAIRY:
○
○
○
○
○
○
○
○
○
○
○
○

MEAT & SEAFOOD:
○
○
○
○
○
○
○
○
○
○
○
○

FRUITS & VEGGIES:
○
○
○
○
○
○
○
○

HERBS & SPICES:
○
○
○
○
○

OTHERS:
○
○
○
○
○
○
○
○
○

GREEN TEA
○
○
○
○
○

NOTES
○
○
○
○
○

WHAT'S FOR TODAY
S
M
T
W
T
F
S

Low Histamine
Grocery List

DATE:

DAIRY:

FRUITS & VEGGIES:

GREEN TEA

NOTES

HERBS & SPICES:

MEAT & SEAFOOD:

OTHERS:

WHAT'S FOR TODAY

S
M
T
W
T
F
S

Low Histamine
Grocery List

DATE:

DAIRY:

FRUITS & VEGGIES:

GREEN TEA

NOTES

HERBS & SPICES:

MEAT & SEAFOOD:

OTHERS:

WHAT'S FOR TODAY

S
M
T
W
T
F
S

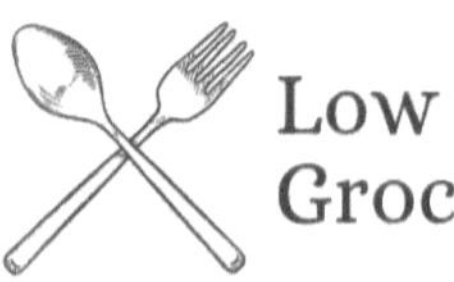

Low Histamine
Grocery List

DATE:

DAIRY:

FRUITS & VEGGIES:

GREEN TEA

NOTES

HERBS & SPICES:

MEAT & SEAFOOD:

OTHERS:

WHAT'S FOR TODAY

S

M

T

W

T

F

S

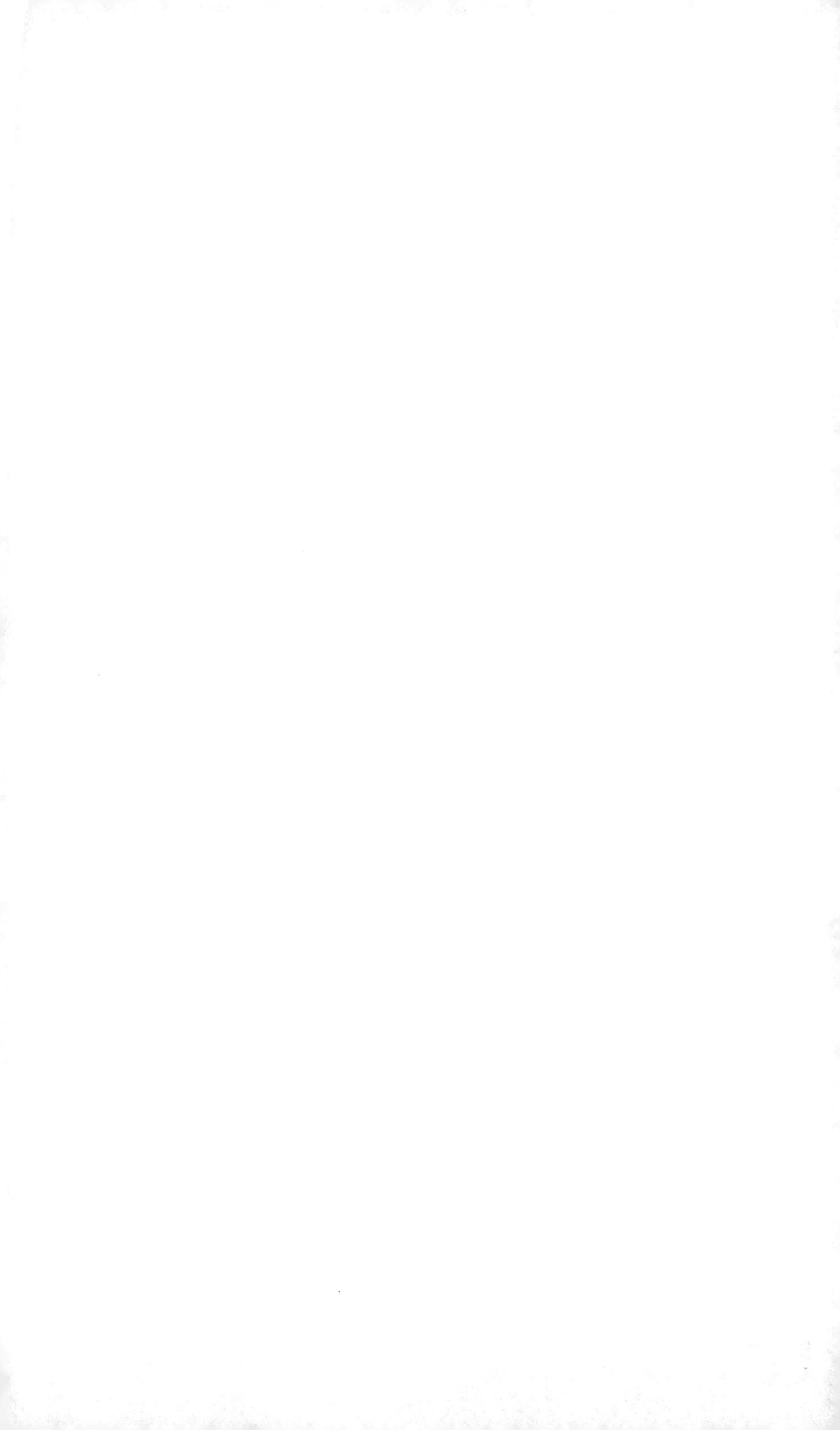

www.ingramcontent.com/pod-product-compliance
Lightning Source LLC
Chambersburg PA
CBHW031311250726
48656CB00005B/1750